Iron Deficiency

*A Patient's Guide to the Most Common
Nutrient Deficiency in the World.*

Joseph J. Shatzel, MD

IRON DEFICIENCY

For my patients.

CONTENTS

ACKNOWLEDGMENTS

Thank you, Tom, Sven, AC, Dave, Erin, and Arjun.

Chapter 1: Introduction

Why are you tired? Iron is vital for the effective production of red blood cells, growth, and development, athletic performance, and overall wellbeing. Even though it plays an important role in our bodies, iron deficiency remains the most common nutrient deficiency in the world.[1] In some countries up to a third of women of childbearing age are iron deficient.[2] Iron deficiency can lead to a multitude of symptoms including anemia, fatigue, difficulty with concentration and productivity, hair thinning and premature hair loss, restless leg syndrome, and a desire to chew on objects like ice or clay. While all of these side effects are reversible when iron deficiency is corrected and the treatment is relatively simple and accessible in some countries, many people remain untreated or inadequately treated. As a hematologist, I believe, as a medical community, we can do better at treating iron deficiency. I am not alone in this belief, as the World Health Organization has made it a priority to reduce the prevalence of anemia in women by 50% before 2025.[2]

I have been trained as a benign hematologist, though the term "benign" is a bit of a misnomer, as there are many illnesses that I treat in my clinical practice that are far from benign. The term refers to the fact that I generally do not treat patients with blood cancers. For decades, in the United States, hematology training has been intertwined with cancer care and most people who train in hematology end up focusing on the treatment of cancers of the blood and other organs. A recent study for example showed that less than 5% of doctors who train in hematology-oncology in America end up treating non-cancerous blood disorders like iron deficiency as the main focus of their practice.[3] There are many layered reasons for this disparity including reimbursement, prestige, and how the training pathway has historically been designed in America. I hope that in the future more trainees will choose to focus on this important field resulting in more treatment innovation and research such that patients with anemia will receive the best evidence-based treatment possible.

One of the largest parts of my practice is helping people with iron deficiency. For instance, my research lab and I published a study involving a greater hospital system in Portland Oregon involving over 400 patients who received intravenous iron in just one year.[4] This number is a small portion of my patient population and it does not include the many patients I treat with oral iron or those we see in follow-up to monitor their iron levels. Most importantly, this number does not reflect the innumerous patients who are never identified, identified, and never followed through on an appointment, or never referred to me.

After seeing many of my patients suffer from iron deficiency, I decided to write this book because I know we can do better. I want to do better. People deserve to have the energy to live their lives, feeling exhausted, being anemic, or even suffering from inadequate treatments for iron deficiency is curable. Many patients I have encountered helped bring me to this conclusion and I will share briefly their stories. Their names have been altered, but their story is true. One such patient, Ava was a 22-year-old college athlete and she was referred to me for iron deficiency. Before I met with her, I reviewed her medical record and it was noted she had been faithfully seeing her primary care doctor every year since she was 18. I noticed that throughout the last 5 years she had been mildly anemic and, in the past, more than one doctor had tried to measure her iron level. Several tests assess how much iron is in the blood, however, the most specific one, the ferritin, had only been sent twice before. In both instances, it was very low. In general, I aim to keep the patient's ferritin over 50 based on studies I outline later in this book, however in her case both times it was <10. Her low ferritin was first noticed about 3 years prior however based on Ava's anemia I could speculate that she had been iron deficient for at least 5 years. Ava had a type of anemia called microcytic anemia. This means that not only was she dealing with too few red blood cells, but that the ones she was making were smaller than normal. This had been noted by at least one doctor prior. She had been recommended to take oral iron tablets. Unfortunately, this has not improved her iron deficiency. She had been taking three pills per day for over a year and this has resulted in daily upset stomach and constipation. She continued to take the iron pills although they were not helping but were making her feel worse. Based on studies I discuss later in this book; you will see that there is no benefit to taking high doses of oral iron. The body will not absorb more than a small amount of iron per day no matter how many pills you take, however, higher doses can worsen symptoms like constipation and upset stomach just like Ava was experiencing.

When I met with Ava, she told me she had felt tired for many years. As a student-athlete, she was already dealing with the extra stresses of early morning workouts and athletic training, not to mention the stressors of taking a full course load. Ava felt like she could not perform at her best in either arena for several years. In short, Ava was tired of being iron deficient.

I prescribed Ava a dose of 1000mg of IV iron to be given in one visit. Some of Ava's doctors had warned her that iron repletion is a slow process that could require as many as 5 infusions but this is simply not true. This misinformation is common and is based on old practices of giving low doses of iron over multiple visits. As outlined later in this book, numerous iron preparations are available in the United States that can safely be given at higher doses requiring only one or two visits.

Six weeks later, I saw Ava in a follow-up visit. She reported feeling much better. Her fatigue had resolved and she reported her athletic performance had improved; she was having an easier time concentrating on her school work. We rechecked her labs and her anemia had resolved.

Her blood counts were now in the normal ranges for the first time in several years, with her ferritin level had risen from <10 to 150. We discussed placing Ava on an iron monitoring protocol so she would not develop an undetectable iron deficiency in the future. I recommended checking her iron levels (the ferritin) 3-4 times per year. If her ferritin decreased to <50, I let her know we could reorder IV iron. Lastly, we discussed why I thought Ava was iron deficient. She described her heavy menstrual cycles for several years. She had what doctors label "heavy menstrual bleeding" or HMB. HMB is a common cause of iron deficiency in younger women. Blood contains a good deal of the body's iron, and each time the body losses some blood iron is lost with it, which on a chronic basis can lead to iron deficiency. I offered to refer Ava to an OB-GYN who specializes in HMB and who could discuss possible treatment options with Ava.

Ava's story is sadly not unique. In nearly every clinic I hold, I meet a new patient who was not expediently referred or treated for their iron deficiency and had evidence of low iron for some time before meeting me. I was glad to have the opportunity to offer her treatments that could improve her quality of life. It is stories like Ava's that inspired me to write this book. No one deserves to chronically have symptoms that are reversible with simple treatments, and as such, I tried to write this book to be accessible, easy to follow, and patient-centered. The ultimate goal of this work is to help patients and their physicians consider and treat their iron deficiency using the best available evidence and treatments.

Chapter 2: How common is iron deficiency?

Iron deficiency is the most common nutrient deficiency in the world.[1] While both men and women can develop iron deficiency, low iron is far more common in women. This is due to the fact that menstruation causes women to lose various amounts of iron each month (as outlined in Chapter 3: What causes iron deficiency). Second, pregnancy and breastfeeding increase a woman's iron needs. Younger, premenopausal women have notable rates of iron deficiency as outlined below. The unfortunate truth is that iron deficiency is more common in underdeveloped countries and the United States certain minorities such as Hispanic and African American women have higher rates of iron deficiency than white women, suggesting there are racial disparities in which women get tested and treated for iron deficiency.[5] Iron deficiency can occur at any age but is most common in women age 12-49.[6] This is particularly of note for pregnant women as iron deficiency is especially prevalent in their age group and can have a negative impact on pregnancy outcomes (as outlined in Chapter 9: Iron deficiency in special populations).

Here are some figures that highlight the high prevalence of iron deficiency:

1. Iron deficiency is the most common cause of anemia in the world.[1]

2. One in five women is iron deficient worldwide (20% of women on the planet).[7]

3. Studies of women of child-bearing age show rates of iron deficiency up to 30-40% depending on the country and age group.[2,8]

4. While more common in younger women some studies have shown up to 12% of older adults are iron deficient.[9]

5. In a study (1960), US college-age women **over half** had iron deficiency based on the most sensitive test (a bone marrow biopsy).[10]

6. Racial and ethnic disparities exist in iron deficiency in the United States and Canada.[5] Here is the incidence of <u>severe</u> iron deficiency in North American women by race based on a large study:
    - Native Americans - 5.2 percent
    - Hispanic Americans – 5.1 percent
    - Black Americans – 4.3 percent

- Pacific Islanders – 3.1 percent
- Asian Americans – 2.1 percent
- White Americans – 2.0 percent

Key Points:

1. Iron deficiency is significantly more common in women
2. Twenty percent of women are iron deficient worldwide
3. Iron deficiency is most prevalent in reproductive age women and pregnant women
4. Racial disparities exist in the prevalence of iron deficiency. Women of color are more likely to be iron deficient than white women.

Chapter 3: What causes iron deficiency?

While there are many possible causes of iron deficiency, there are three main categories to consider as to why people are iron deficient 1) You are losing iron due to blood loss. Blood loss is by far the most common category, 2) You are not absorbing iron due to a problem in your gastrointestinal system, and 3) You are not taking in enough iron. The last category is the least common cause by far in the adult patients I treat. However, it should be noted, it may be more common in other countries. In the following chapter, we have broken down the various causes of iron deficiency into these three categories. A final category is iron deficiency secondary intense exercise. This is a rare cause of iron deficiency outlined at the end of this chapter.

1) Iron deficiency secondary to blood loss.

A good deal of the body's iron is stored in the blood. This is because iron is one of the key components of red blood cells and is used to make hemoglobin, a chemical that helps red blood cells carry oxygen to different parts of the body and remove carbon dioxide. For example, every time someone donates a unit of blood they also give 200-250mg of iron along with it.[11] It should be no surprise then that bleeding can cause iron deficiency as iron is both lost as blood exits the body and consumed as the body tries to manufacture new red blood cells.

Chronic small amounts of blood loss can outpace the amount of iron the body absorbs and lead to iron deficiency. This is most commonly seen in the following conditions:

Common causes of blood loss that can lead to iron deficiency:

1. *Menstrual blood losses.* The spectrum of normal menstruation to heavy menstrual bleeding (HMB) can be the cause of, or contribute to, iron deficiency.
2. *Bleeding from the stomach or esophagus.* This can include stomach ulcers, chronic irritation of the esophagus (esophagitis), and sometimes when the stomach moves into an unintended section of the body, this is referred to as a hiatal hernia and can cause chronic bleeding and iron deficiency. Stomach and esophagus cancers are not common, and they can also cause bleeding and iron deficiency. People who take regular doses of

Ibuprofen or who drink alcohol heavily can develop a stomach ulcer or have a bleed from the upper gastrointestinal tract; it is something doctors may inquire about when considering the cause of your iron deficiency.

3. *Bleeding from the colon.* This can be secondary to issues in the colon that cause bleeding such as arteriovenous malformations (AVM), which are abnormal blood vessels that can cause bleeding diverticulosis (outpouching in the colon that can cause bleeding), or rarely colon cancer. This is the reason iron-deficient patients are sometimes sent for a colonoscopy, to look for any of these causes of iron deficiency. A very rare cause is inflammatory bowel diseases like Crohn's disease or ulcerative colitis.

2) You are not absorbing iron due to a problem in your gastrointestinal system:

Iron is absorbed in the upper part of the gastrointestinal (GI) tract in a section known as the duodenum.[2] The duodenum is part of the small intestine, just after the stomach and it is not uncommon that diseases that irritate the stomach or duodenum can lead to iron deficiency. This is a side effect for people who have had a gastric bypass or they have celiac disease. People who have had a gastric bypass may need periodic iron repletion as they can chronically be iron deficient due to poor absorption.

3) You are not taking in enough iron:

As a doctor practicing in the United States, I can honestly say that I have never encountered a patient whose diet was the sole cause of their iron deficiency. While not generally the sole cause, a diet with modest iron content can worsen iron deficiency in patients who are bleeding or had a problem absorbing iron. Vegetarians have higher rates of iron deficiency, for instance, suggesting that eating meat may improve iron stores and that iron from certain food sources can have diminished absorption.[12] More information on iron and diet is listed in Chapter 7: How is iron deficiency treated.

4) Additional considerations

Exercise-induced iron deficiency:

Some studies have suggested elite runners and triathletes have high rates of iron deficiency.[13] While the cause of exercise-induced iron deficiency is not entirely known, it may be secondary to increased iron needs, decreased absorption due to inflammation, or blood breakdown from exercise. This phenomenon is unlikely to occur in people who exercise moderately. Strenuous repetitive exercise in studies of military recruits showed that young healthy males participating in prolonged strenuous training programs can develop iron deficiency; at the 15-month follow-up, 29% had developed new-onset iron deficiency anemia and 65% showed evidence of iron deficiency.[14]

Iron Deficiency in Children:

There are some unique considerations that are different than adults when it comes to iron deficiency in children. There is a separate section on iron deficiency in children (as outlined in Chapter 9: Iron deficiency in special populations). In brief, if children are fed cow's milk before one year of age, they can develop iron deficiency secondary to irritation of the gastrointestinal tract and subsequent bleeding. Likewise, older children who drink excessive amounts of cow's milk can also develop iron deficiency due to similarly gastrointestinal irritation and the low iron content in a cow milk-based diet. While formula-based milk is iron-fortified, children who receive breast milk for an extended period or who were born prematurely may benefit from iron supplementation.

Table 1: Causes of iron deficiency

Issue	Affected Organ(s)	Symptoms leading to Iron Deficiency
Blood loss	Uterus (menstruation)	Heavy menstrual bleeding
	Stomach/ Esophagus	Stomach ulcers Chronic irritation of esophagus Hiatal hernia
	Colon	Arteriovenous malformation Bleeding diverticulosis
Lack of Iron Absorption	Gastrointestinal	Diseases that irritate stomach or duodenum Side effect of gastric bypass and celiac disease
Lack of Iron in Diet		Very rare Modest iron consumption can worsen deficiency in individuals with bleeding or issues with absorption of iron

Key Points:

1. The most common cause of iron deficiency is blood loss, with menstrual blood loss or bleeding from the gastrointestinal tract being the most common causes.
2. Less commonly, disorders of the gastrointestinal system that prevent absorption can cause iron deficiency, such as undergoing a gastric bypass or having celiac disease.
3. While rare in the United States, and unlikely to be the sole cause of iron deficiency, a low iron diet can precipitate or worsen iron deficiency.
4. A consideration for children, milk intake is a risk factor for iron deficiency in children.

Chapter 4: How is iron deficiency diagnosed?

The diagnosis of iron deficiency can be confusing as there is more than one laboratory test to look for iron deficiency. When doing the assessment for iron deficiency, I consider the following labs:

1. Complete blood count (CBC)
2. Ferritin
3. Serum Iron and Total Iron Binding Capacity (TIBC)
4. % Iron Saturation

The complete blood count (CBC). The CBC is looking at all the cells in the blood and specifically the white blood cell count (WBC), the relative amount of red blood cells (this is listed as hemoglobin or hematocrit), and the platelet count. The CBC is used to diagnose anemia which is a common complication of iron deficiency. The best test to diagnose anemia is hemoglobin. If the hemoglobin is low, you are anemic. The hematocrit is another way to measure hemoglobin. Anemia caused by iron deficiency, if severe, tends to make small red blood cells. This is called "microcytic anemia." The best test to measure red blood cell size is called the mean corpuscular volume or "MCV" If you have low hemoglobin and low MCV you have microcytic anemia and likely have iron deficiency.

- Low hemoglobin is called anemia
- Low MCV and low hemoglobin means you have "microcytic anemia"
- The most common cause of microcytic anemia is iron deficiency

Ferritin. If you could only get one test to see if someone is iron deficient it would be the ferritin. A ferritin > 50 essentially rules out iron deficiency. The is the test I focus on when trying to assess if a patient is iron deficient. I have made a ferritin of 50 as a cut-off for ruling out iron deficiency as studies that used the most sensitive test (a bone marrow biopsy) found this level all but rules out iron deficiency.

> **Why is a ferritin of 50 the cut-off for treatment?** Studies of iron deficiency have not been consistent on the cut-off to determine if someone is iron deficient. In my practice, we use a ferritin of 50 because 2 studies showed that treating women with a ferritin <50 improved their symptoms.[15-17]

Serum Iron and Total Iron Binding Capacity (TIBC). These tests can be confusing, and to be honest, they are not as useful as the ferritin. For the purposes of diagnosing iron deficiency focus on the ferritin.

% Iron Saturation. This test is also of limited utility and can be altered if someone ate a high iron meal just before the test. If the % iron saturation is low and the ferritin is high that can be a sign of inflammation (sometimes called inflammatory anemia or anemia of chronic disease).

Table 2: Lab findings in iron deficiency and what they mean.

Tests for Iron Deficiency	What is being measured	Results interpretation
Complete blood count (CBC)	Hemoglobin concentration	Low hemoglobin concentration – Anemia
	RBC size through measuring MCV	Low MCV and low hemoglobin – "microcytic anemia"
Ferritin	Ferritin concentration	Greater than 50 – no iron deficiency Less than 50 – potential iron deficiency
Serum Iron Total Iron Binding Capacity (TIBC)	not most helpful (focus on ferritin)	*not the most helpful
% Iron Saturation	Iron concentration	Low % saturation and high ferritin is a sign of inflammatory anemia

Key Points:

1. Ferritin is the best test to see if you are iron deficient
2. If you have a ferritin <50 studies show you may benefit from treatment
3. If your ferritin is >50 and you are symptomatic, something else is causing your anemia or symptoms
4. The other tests (serum iron, TIBC, % saturation) are generally are not needed to see if you are iron deficient.

Chapter 5: What are the stages of iron deficiency?

Iron deficiency is a spectrum from mildly decreased ferritin to severe anemia. It is important to point out that even the early stages of iron deficiency have been shown to cause clinical symptoms that can improve with iron repletion (a point that many doctors overlook). In this chapter, we will discuss the two stages of iron deficiency.

Stage 1. Latent Iron Deficiency (Ferritin <50, normal Hemoglobin). Latent iron deficiency occurs when people have low iron but have not yet developed anemia. Many studies suggest this is the most common form of iron deficiency.[18] There are two things to remember about latent iron deficiency. 1) it is common and 2) it causes symptoms that can be reversed with iron repletion.

How common is latent iron deficiency? This varies based on the study, however, in some studies over half of the women have latent iron deficiency.[18] Studies in Indian nursing students found a 27.5% rate of latent iron deficiency.[8,17] Studies in athletes have also found high rates in female athletes (26%) as compared to male athletes (11%).[19]

What are the symptoms of latent iron deficiency? Despite how common it is, affecting a quarter or more of younger women in certain studies, there are relatively few studies looking at the clinical effects of latent iron deficiency. A handful of studies have described a measurable effect on vitality, energy, and concentration from correcting latent iron deficiency. Two clinical trials found measurable improvements in fatigue.[8,16] Another small study found that correction of latent Iron deficiency improved cognitive function.[20] Other studies noted reduced endurance, sensation-seeking behavior, low brain activity in the front part of the brain, increased withdrawal tendencies, and decreased motivation and fatigue in women with latent iron deficiency.[21]

Stage 2. Iron Deficiency Anemia. Iron deficiency anemia is present when a person's ferritin is <50 and their hemoglobin or hematocrit is below the normal range for their sex. As mentioned previously, the type of anemia that is caused by iron deficiency is called "microcytic anemia" which means the red blood cells are smaller than normal. The lab that measures red blood cell size is called the "mean corpuscular volume" or "MCV." Not every case of iron deficiency will have a low MCV. It can be normal and this is called "normocytic anemia."

There are a few things to know about iron deficiency anemia listed below that will be expanded on in the next few chapters:

1. Iron deficiency anemia can cause multiple symptoms including fatigue, low motivation, hair thinning, restless leg syndrome, and a desire to chew on ice or clay.
2. There are essentially two medical treatments for iron deficiency anemia:
    a. oral iron
    b. intravenous (IV) iron

Your doctor will also consider why you have iron deficiency anemia (as outlined in Chapter 3: What causes iron deficiency) and may be able to offer some treatment to prevent iron deficiency in the future.

Lastly, if your iron deficiency anemia is very severe your doctor may need to give you a blood transfusion. This is not common in patients who are seen in the clinic, however in some severe cases involving bleeding from the GI tract patients may need to be admitted to the hospital and given blood transfusions along with other treatments.

Key Points:

1. Iron deficiency without anemia (latent iron deficiency) is common and can cause symptoms that are improved with iron repletion.
2. Later stages of iron deficiency will result in anemia.

Chapter 6: What are the symptoms of iron deficiency?

Iron deficiency can lead to multiple symptoms. In my medical practice, I have encountered a wide range of symptoms from mild fatigue, to patients with severe anemia who were literally unable to function. The symptoms tend to track with the level of iron deficiency and the level of anemia. This is not a hard and fast rule however and I have worked with patients who had mild iron deficiency based on lab work, but significant symptoms that resolved after iron repletion. Some patients did not even realize they had symptoms until they underwent iron repletion and experienced improvement in their energy and vigor. In the following chapter, I have endeavored to outline all the possible symptoms of iron deficiency and the relevant studies the inform doctors and patients about iron deficiency.

1. **Fatigue.** Fatigue is the most common side effect I hear patients report from their iron deficiency. This symptom can range from subtle (i.e., barely

noticeable) to debilitating in older patients with significant iron deficiency anemia.

2. **Poor Concentration.** Younger women with good iron stores perform better on cognitive tasks and test speed than iron-deficient women. Treatment of iron deficiency resulted in a 5–7-fold improvement in cognitive performance and improved speed in completing cognitive tasks.[22]

3. **Pale skin.** Doctors call this "pallor" and its call be seen with anemia in general. As anemia becomes more severe the likelihood of pallor increases.

4. **Hair Thinning.** While somewhat controversial, many experts believe that iron deficiency contributes to certain types of hair loss and that correcting iron deficiency improves hair thinning and loss.[23]

5. **Restless leg syndrome.** Multiple studies have suggested that correcting iron deficiency improves restless leg syndrome.[24]

6. **Spooning of the fingernails.** Changes in the fingernails can be seen with iron deficiency. This is referred to by doctors as "koilonychia."

7. **Exercise intolerance.** As previously described in this book, strenuous repetitive exercise can cause iron deficiency. This has been shown in studies of military recruits involving young healthy males participating in prolonged strenuous training programs; at the 15-month follow-up, 29% of participants had developed new-onset iron deficiency anemia and 65% showed evidence of iron deficiency.[14] Ironically as iron levels get lower

one's athletic performance decreases. There have been numerous studies on the effects of iron supplementation worthy of discussion. As an example, one group of scientists analyzed 22 clinical studies that looked at the effects of oral iron supplementation on athletic performance in iron-deficient women. They found that iron supplementation improved athletic performance by several measurements including both maximal and submaximal exercise performance as demonstrated by a lower heart rate and oxygen intake required to achieve defined workloads.[25]

8. **A desire to chew on non-food objects such as ice or clay.** This is known as "pica" and is not an uncommon side effect seen in patients with iron deficiency. When the desire is focused around chewing on ice the medical term is called "pagophagia." The desire to chew on ice and other substances can quickly stop after a person's iron deficiency is treated.[26]

9. **Red urine after eating beets.** This is known as "beeturia" and yes, this is a real thing that happens to people with iron deficiency. In fact, beeturia occurs in 50-80% of people with iron deficiency.[27] Beeturia is believed to be caused by certain pigments in beets that are broken down by iron. If your system is low on iron the pigments are not broken down, there is a red tint to the urine.

10. **Hearing loss.** This complication of iron deficiency is not fully understood and it is unclear how much iron deficiency is a risk factor for hearing loss if it is a risk factor at all. One study of 305,339 patients found a high rate of hearing loss

in iron-deficient patients vs those who were not iron deficient (1.6% vs 0.7%).[28]

Rare complications of iron deficiency:

Plummer-Vinson syndrome (PVS). PVS is a very rare syndrome that tended to occur in women nearing menopause. The syndrome is characterized by severe iron deficiency, difficulty swallowing due to the development of webs in the esophagus, and inflammation of the tongue (this is call glossitis) and the lips (this is called cheilitis).

Chlorosis. Chlorosis is an antiquated term that was previously used to describe the very severe iron deficiency in younger premenopausal women. This term (and the very severe forms of iron deficiency anemia it described) is not commonly used or seen today. The word "chlorosis" derives from the observation that the skin of younger people with chronic severe iron deficiency anemia developed a green hue.[29] This finding is not routinely encountered these days due to improved medical care and early detection of iron deficiency anemia.

Key Points:

1. Iron deficiency can cause numerous symptoms
2. Common symptoms like fatigue, exercise intolerance, and trouble concentrating can be reversed with treatment.

Chapter 7: How is iron deficiency treated?

In general, there are three main ways to treat iron deficiency: 1) dietary interventions, 2) oral iron, and 3) intravenous (IV) iron. In rare cases, a patient may be severely anemic and a blood transfusion would also be considered on a case-by-case basis, a fourth possible treatment used only in severe circumstances. The important thing to take away from this chapter is that IV iron is the most effective way to treat iron deficiency. Oral iron and dietary interventions are effective in some patients but are generally less likely to be successful. In the following chapter, we outline what you need to know about each therapy and our preferred method of deciding which therapy is best for each patient.

1). Dietary interventions. It is very rare for adults in resource-rich countries to be iron deficient due solely to poor iron intake from their diet. Many foods such as cereals and grains are iron-fortified in the United States, helping to ensure enough iron is consumed in modern societies. Nearly all adults that are iron deficient are so due to blood loss or poor iron absorption. As outlined in Chapter 9, in this book, children who are maintained on a cow-milk-heavy diet can develop iron deficiency, and thus considering this dietary intervention can lead to improvements in children. In adults, changes in diet can have a small impact on iron stores. This is illustrated by the fact that those who keep a vegan diet are more likely to be iron deficient than those who choose to eat meat.[30]

While I do have many patients ask me about changing their diet to help treat their iron deficiency, I counsel them that dietary changes are unlikely to make a significant impact on their iron levels. Nevertheless, I do counsel on the types of dietary iron, such as heme-based iron in meats and non-heme irons found in dairy, eggs, and various plants in our diet. Heme-based iron is more readily aborded and given this if eating meat is within your personal preferences it can help increase the iron content in your diet.

For those who wish to be conscious of the iron content in their diet here is a list of iron-rich foods:

Table 3: Iron content in common foods.[31]

Types of Food	Food Product	Serving Size	Iron Content
Vegetables / plants	Spinach	3.5 oz (100 grams)	2.71 mg
	Potato	1 potato (213 grams)	1.72 mg
	Broccoli	1 cup (156 grams)	1.05 mg
	Green beans	1 cup (100 grams)	1.03 mg
Meats	Eggs	1 egg (50 grams)	0.84 mg
	Organ meats	3.5 oz (100 grams)	6.54 mg
	Turkey (dark meat)	3.5 oz (100 grams)	1.43 mg
	Red meat (ground beef)	3.5 oz (100 grams)	2.74 mg
Legumes/ other	Quinoa	1 cup (185 grams)	2.76 mg

	Lentils	1 cup (198 grams)	6.59 mg
	Rye bread	1 slice (32 grams)	0.906 mg
	Tofu	0.5 cups (126 grams)	3.35 mg
Seafood	Fish	3 oz (85 grams)	1.40 mg
	Clams	3 oz (85 gram)	2.39 mg

2). Oral Iron: Oral iron is the most commonly used means to treat iron deficiency and is usually the first treatment attempted to address iron deficiency. Unfortunately for many patients, oral iron is not completely effective in all patients and it can lead to some unwanted side effects such as constipation or upset stomach. For these reasons, we generally trial oral iron for 8-12 weeks in our patients. If the ferritin has not increased to over 50 with an 8-12 week trial of oral iron, or if intolerable side effects occur we generally stop oral iron and offer IV Iron.

How should oral iron be taken and which formulation should you choose?

There is no consensus on the best dose of oral iron. In general, only 10-40% of the iron taken into the stomach is absorbed, and even with high doses of oral iron (200 mg), only 10-60 mg is absorbed into the system.[32] Given this, any formulation of iron with at least 60 mg of iron is likely sufficient. Generally, in the over-the-counter iron preparation, this is equivalent to one tablet or a single dose of liquid iron preparation. There is no benefit to adding more tablets or taking tablets twice a day since the stomach will not absorb more iron. I have unfortunately seen many patients try to take iron tablets several times per day which had no effect on their iron levels but led to unnecessary constipation.

1. Any preparation of oral iron that has more than 60 mg of iron is sufficient.
2. **Only one dose per day is needed.** There is no benefit to adding more tablets or taking tablets twice a day.
3. If daily dosing is causing too many side effects taking the pill **every other day** is fine. Several

studies have shown this is an effective way to take oral iron. [33]

4. Some studies suggest taking oral iron with Vitamin C will improve absorption. Some patients choose to take it with orange juice, others use vitamin C tablets.
5. Avoid taking your oral iron with coffee, tea, or milk which can limit its absorption.

What are the side effects of oral iron?

Unfortunately, certain patients experience unwanted side effects from oral iron. In clinical trials of oral iron, about one in three patients will report a side effect.[34,35] The rates of side effects in clinical trials vary somewhat based on the type of iron used, the dose of iron, and the population being studied. A rough estimate of the most common side effects is described below:

- Dark-colored stools (~30%)
- Constipation (~20%)
- Diarrhea (~20%)
- Abdominal pain (~5-10%)
- Nausea (~5-10%)

No one deserves to feel poorly from their treatment. When I care for patients who have significant side effects from oral iron, I consider switching to IV iron. Other alternatives include 1) switching your dose to every other day if you are not trying that already or 2) trying a different formulation of oral iron. My preference is to switch to IV iron in truly intolerant people. In the next section, you will see that IV iron is more likely to effectively raise ferritin.

How often does oral iron effectively raise the ferritin to over 50?

IV iron does a better job of reversing iron deficiency than oral iron. That said, oral iron is effective in about one in four patients at reversing iron deficiency from gastrointestinal blood loss (25%).[34] On average oral iron will increase the ferritin level by about 11 points at 12 weeks.[16]

Who should avoid oral iron and instead be treated directly with IV Iron: The following groups of patients will not do well with oral iron and should preferentially be treated with IV iron upfront:

- Individuals who failed to get their ferritin over 50 with oral iron or those who were intolerant to oral
- Patients who have had a gastric bypass or similar stomach surgery
- Patients with celiac disease
- Patients with inflammatory bowel disease (e.g., ulcerative colitis, Crone's disease, ctc).
- Pregnant women in the latter half of pregnancy
- Patients with kidney disease on hemodialysis

3). IV Iron: IV Iron is more effective and quicker than oral iron at reversing iron deficiency, and it does not cause chronic side effects as oral iron may when taken long term. IV iron is given directly into the vein, usually at an infusion clinic. There are multiple types available for your doctor to choose from. There is one key point to keep in mind:

1. Your doctor should select a type of iron and dose that can be given in one or two visits. There are some older formulations of iron that require up to 5 visits to get a full dose and there is no benefit to using those products.

Here is a list of the different iron preparations available and the usual dose is given:

Table 4: IV Iron formulations[36]

Drug Name (generic)	Approved dose	Commonly used doses	Infusion time
LMW iron dextran	100 mg per dose	1000 mg	1 h
Ferumoxytol	510 mg over 15 min	510 mg x 2	15 min
Ferric carboxymaltose	750 mg over 15 min	750 mg x 2	15 min
Iron isomaltoside	20 mg/kg (1000 mg if >66 kg)	1000 mg	15 min
Iron sucrose		200 – 300 mg	15 min
Sodium ferric Gluconate		125 – 187.5 mg	1 h

What are the side effects of IV Iron?

Side effects are not common with IV iron and tend to occur during the infusion if they are going to occur. As part of my research group, we published a study looking at over 900 doses of IV Iron and found that relevant side effects occurred in <3% of patients.[4] In our experience, 97% of patients have mild or no side effects from IV iron. Rarely, patients can experience the side effects below:

1. Minor infusions reactions can happen during the infusion (e.g., mild flushing, muscle/joint ache, chest tightness). These reactions are rare and tend to be short-lived. If reactions like this occur, they usually go away quickly, especially if the infusion is paused.
2. Severe reactions that require a medical evaluation are extremely rare (<1%).[37]

How Effective is IV Iron?

IV iron is more likely to correct iron deficiency than oral iron and it works much faster. In a large clinical study, our research group reported in 2020 the average increase in ferritin after a single dose of IV iron was 70-80 ng/dl.[4] Similarly, a study comparing IV iron to oral iron found that IV iron corrected about 75% of patients with iron deficiency while oral iron was only effective about 25% of the time.

Key Points:

Diet:

1. Dietary changes alone are unlikely to fully correct iron deficiency.

Oral iron:

1. Any preparation of oral iron that has more than 60 mg of iron is sufficient.
2. **Only one dose per day is needed.** There is no benefit to adding more tablets or taking tablets twice a day.
3. If daily dosing is causing too many side effects taking the pill **every other day** is fine. Several studies have shown this is an effective way to take oral iron. [33]
4. Some studies suggest taking oral iron with Vitamin C will improve absorption. Some patients choose to take it with orange juice, while others use vitamin C tablets.
5. Avoid taking your oral iron with coffee, tea, or milk which can limit its absorption.
6. Patients should be given a trial of oral iron for 8-12 weeks. If ferritin does not increase to 50 at that time or significant side effects occur then IV iron should be considered.

IV Iron:

1. Your doctor should select a type of iron and dose that can be given in one or two visits. There are some older formulations of iron that require up to 5 visits to get a full dose and there is no benefit to using those products.

Chapter 8: How is iron deficiency prevented in the future?

A common question we get from patients who have successfully had their iron deficiency treated is how to prevent it in the future.

1. **Monitoring for recurrent iron deficiency.** There is no clear-cut guideline on how often to monitor iron levels after a person has been successfully treated for iron deficiency. I tend to tailor to plan based on the cause of iron deficiency. For instance, if patients were iron deficient from a single episode of gastrointestinal bleeding that has resolved then it may be appropriate to not routinely check ferritin. On the other hand, patients who are iron deficient from persistent heavy menstrual bleeding tend to benefit from routine monitoring as their ferritin is likely to decrease again after treatment of iron deficiency. In such patients, I tend to check ferritin every 4-6 months depending on the situation and reinitiate iron if the ferritin is <50.

The figure below outlines our usual monitoring protocol in patients who have continued blood loss or poor iron absorption (e.g., such as patients with a history of gastric surgery).

Figure 1. How to Monitor Iron:

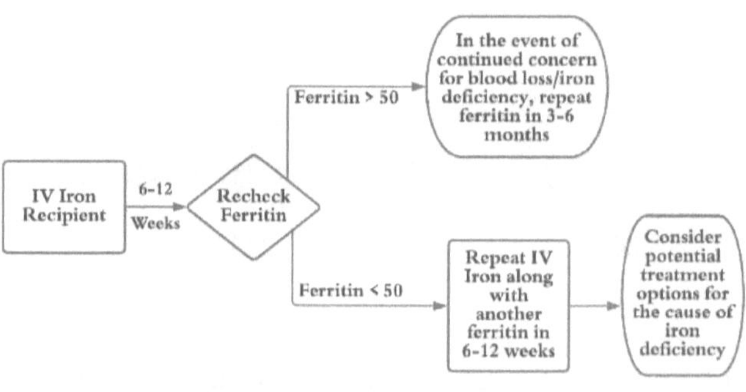

2. **Treating the cause of iron deficiency.** For patients who have iron deficiency due to blood loss (i.e., heavy menstrual bleeding or gastrointestinal bleeding), there are likely treatment options that could help limit or stop your bleeding. Ask your primary care doctor or OB-GYN about medical therapies that could help. Some examples of options that could be considered if they align with your treatment goals are listed below:

Treatment options for heavy menstrual bleeding:

- Oral Contraceptive Pills
- Intrauterine contraceptive devices (IUD)

- Medicines to help prevent the breakdown of blood clots (i.e., antifibrinolytic drugs such as Tranexamic Acid)
- Surgical treatments that your OB-GYN may offer in select circumstances

Treatment options for gastrointestinal bleeding:

- For bleeding from the stomach or esophagus, your doctor may offer drugs to lower the acidity of the stomach (these are called proton pump inhibitors (PPI) of histidine receptor antagonists (H2RA)).

- If your gastroenterologist chooses to do a colonoscopy or endoscopy of your stomach there are several local techniques they can use to treat and prevent bleeding.

3. **Is there a benefit to continued oral iron?** Many patients who tried to deplete their iron levels with oral iron unsuccessfully, and who ultimately go on to receive IV iron, ask about continuing oral iron. In general, if oral iron causes side effects such as upset stomach or constipation it is not worth continuing. Likewise, if oral iron had no impact on your ferritin levels there is not much utility in continuing it. Here are some key points:

- If you previously tried oral iron and it was not effective, or caused significant symptoms, and you had a good response to IV iron, generally we recommend stopping oral iron and proceeding with IV iron again if your iron deficiency relapses.
- If oral iron worked well for you, or you had a bad experience with IV iron and do not wish to continue it, continuing oral iron once a day or every other day is reasonable. Many clinical studies suggest that intermittent oral iron prevents anemia and iron deficiency in adolescent and premenopausal women.[38]

Key points:

1. For patients with ongoing blood loss, it is reasonable to recheck ferritin periodically after their iron deficiency is corrected. Treatment can be reinitiated if ferritin drops to <50 in the future.
2. If you did not respond to oral iron previously or if you developed any significant side effects then generally, we do not continue it.

Chapter 9: Iron deficiency in special populations.

The preceding chapters of this book outlined what the medical community knows about iron deficiency in general. The most common population of patients who experience iron deficiency are premenopausal women, and as such a good proportion of the research on iron deficiency focuses on this population. There are some other groups of patients however that deserve special attention due to considerations around their iron deficiency and its treatment. In the following section, we outline important information on the management of iron deficiency in children, pregnancy, and patients with heart disease or kidney failure.

Children: Iron deficiency occurs in approximately 7% of American children, however, rates are much higher in resource-poor countries.[39] The causes of iron deficiency in children are varied, however, they include maternal iron deficiency, premature birth, and poor dietary intake of iron. Specifically, if children are feed cow's milk before one year of age, they can develop iron deficiency secondary to irritation of the gastrointestinal tract and subsequent bleeding. Likewise, older children who drink excessive amounts of cow's milk can also develop iron deficiency due to similarly gastrointestinal irritation and the low iron content in a cow milk-based diet. While formula-based milk is iron-fortified, children who receive breast milk for an extended period or who were born prematurely are at risk for iron deficiency and may benefit from iron supplementation.

Heart failure: Several trials have looked at the benefit of IV Iron in patients with heart failure and a ferritin <100. One study found that IV iron reduced the risk of heart failure hospitalizations.[40] Similar trials in patients with heart failure have found that IV iron improves symptoms, functional capacity, and quality of life.[41] Given these positive findings patients with certain types of heart failure are often offered IV iron by their doctor.

Kidney Failure: Patients with kidney failure often suffer from anemia. The kidneys produce a hormone (erythropoietin) that functions in red blood cell production. Patients with renal failure often have significant anemia. Such patients are often treated with higher doses of IV iron than the general population and often given injections of erythropoietin to help treat their anemia.

Pregnancy: Iron deficiency is common in pregnancy. This is due to both the fact that iron deficiency is common in younger women for all the reasons outlined in this book, and that pregnancy requires extra iron intake to help create blood cells for the developing baby. In fact, iron needs can go up by 4-6 fold during the later trimesters of pregnancy.[42] Typically all pregnant women are given oral iron, often in the form of prenatal vitamins, to prevent iron deficiency. Pregnant women are often screened for iron deficiency when first establishing with their pregnancy care team, especially if they are notably anemic. The treatment of iron deficiency in pregnancy is similar to the treatment in general with some notable exceptions.

1. Oral iron is generally tried first as long as women can tolerate it. Oral iron can cause GI upset and constipation, both of which may be already present in pregnancy. One important point is that IV iron is generally avoided in the first trimester of pregnancy, and as such oral iron may be the only option early in pregnancy.
2. IV iron is typically used in pregnant women who have significant side effects or who do not respond to oral iron as long as they are in their second or third trimester. There are specific formulations your doctor may select in pregnancy as some formulations are more studied than others in pregnant women.

Conclusion:

I hope this book has been useful to you and your loved ones who may be dealing with iron deficiency. Low iron is common in younger women and the high prevalence described in this book highlights that we can do better as a medical community at identifying and treating iron deficiency. Aside from anemia, iron deficiency causes a variety of symptoms that can be reversed with proper treatment. Oral iron can be useful in certain circumstances; however, intravenous iron tends to be more effective and can be a useful treatment in those who do not respond to oral iron or who have side effects from its use. If you have questions that were not addressed by this book or wish to learn more about iron deficiency, as always, you should speak with your primary care doctor or hematologist.

Be well.

References:

1. Global, regional, and national incidence, prevalence, and years lived with disability for 328 diseases and injuries for 195 countries, 1990-2016: a systematic analysis for the Global Burden of Disease Study 2016. *Lancet*. Sep 16 2017;390(10100):1211-1259.
2. Pasricha SR, Tye-Din J, Muckenthaler MU, Swinkels DW. Iron deficiency. *Lancet*. Jan 16 2021;397(10270):233-248.
3. Masselink LE, Erikson CE, Connell NT, et al. Associations between hematology/oncology fellows' training and mentorship experiences and hematology-only career plans. *Blood Adv*. Nov 12 2019;3(21):3278-3286.
4. Cohen J, Khudanyan A, Lu J, et al. A multicenter study evaluating the effectiveness and safety of single-dose low molecular weight iron dextran vs single-dose ferumoxytol for the treatment of iron deficiency. *Am J Hematol*. Dec 2020;95(12):1572-1577.
5. Barton JC, Wiener HH, Acton RT, et al. Prevalence of iron deficiency in 62,685 women of seven race/ethnicity groups: The HEIRS Study. *PLoS One*. 2020;15(4):e0232125.
6. Iron deficiency--United States, 1999-2000. *MMWR Morb Mortal Wkly Rep*. Oct 11 2002;51(40):897-899.
7. Kassebaum NJ, Jasrasaria R, Naghavi M, et al. A systematic analysis of global anemia burden from 1990 to 2010. *Blood*. Jan 30 2014;123(5):615-624.
8. Mehta BC. Iron deficiency amongst nursing students. *Indian J Med Sci*. Sep 2004;58(9):389-393.

9. Price EA, Mehra R, Holmes TH, Schrier SL. Anemia in older persons: etiology and evaluation. *Blood Cells Mol Dis.* Feb 15 2011;46(2):159-165.

10. Scott DE, Pritchard JA. Iron deficiency in healthy young college women. *Jama.* Mar 20 1967;199(12):897-900.

11. Remacha A, Sanz C, Contreras E, et al. Guidelines on haemovigilance of post-transfusional iron overload. *Blood Transfus.* Jan 2013;11(1):128-139.

12. Haider LM, Schwingshackl L, Hoffmann G, Ekmekcioglu C. The effect of vegetarian diets on iron status in adults: A systematic review and meta-analysis. *Crit Rev Food Sci Nutr.* May 24 2018;58(8):1359-1374.

13. Coates A, Mountjoy M, Burr J. Incidence of Iron Deficiency and Iron Deficient Anemia in Elite Runners and Triathletes. *Clin J Sport Med.* Sep 2017;27(5):493-498.

14. Epstein D, Borohovitz A, Merdler I, et al. Prevalence of Iron Deficiency and Iron Deficiency Anemia in Strenuously Training Male Army Recruits. *Acta Haematol.* 2018;139(3):141-147.

15. DeLoughery TG. Microcytic anemia. *N Engl J Med.* Dec 25 2014;371(26):2537.

16. Vaucher P, Druais PL, Waldvogel S, Favrat B. Effect of iron supplementation on fatigue in nonanemic menstruating women with low ferritin: a randomized controlled trial. *Cmaj.* Aug 7 2012;184(11):1247-1254.

17. Verdon F, Burnand B, Stubi CL, et al. Iron supplementation for unexplained fatigue in non-anaemic women: double blind randomised placebo controlled trial. *Bmj.* May 24 2003;326(7399):1124.

18. Abuaisha M, Itani H, El Masri R, Antoun J. Prevalence of Iron Deficiency (ID) without anemia in the general population presenting to

primary care clinics: a cross-sectional study. *Postgrad Med.* Apr 2020;132(3):282-287.

19. Malczewska J, Szczepańska B, Stupnicki R, Sendecki W. The assessment of frequency of iron deficiency in athletes from the transferrin receptor-ferritin index. *Int J Sport Nutr Exerc Metab.* Mar 2001;11(1):42-52.

20. Leonard AJ, Chalmers KA, Collins CE, Patterson AJ. A study of the effects of latent iron deficiency on measures of cognition: a pilot randomised controlled trial of iron supplementation in young women. *Nutrients.* Jun 23 2014;6(6):2419-2435.

21. Dziembowska I, Kwapisz J, Izdebski P, Żekanowska E. Mild iron deficiency may affect female endurance and behavior. *Physiol Behav.* Jun 1 2019;205:44-50.

22. Murray-Kolb LE, Beard JL. Iron treatment normalizes cognitive functioning in young women. *Am J Clin Nutr.* Mar 2007;85(3):778-787.

23. Trost LB, Bergfeld WF, Calogeras E. The diagnosis and treatment of iron deficiency and its potential relationship to hair loss. *J Am Acad Dermatol.* May 2006;54(5):824-844.

24. Trotti LM, Becker LA. Iron for the treatment of restless legs syndrome. *Cochrane Database Syst Rev.* Jan 4 2019;1(1):Cd007834.

25. Pasricha SR, Low M, Thompson J, Farrell A, De-Regil LM. Iron supplementation benefits physical performance in women of reproductive age: a systematic review and meta-analysis. *J Nutr.* Jun 2014;144(6):906-914.

26. Osman YM, Wali YA, Osman OM. Craving for ice and iron-deficiency anemia: a case series from Oman. *Pediatr Hematol Oncol.* Mar 2005;22(2):127-131.

27. Sotos JG. Beeturia and iron absorption. *Lancet.* Sep 18 1999;354(9183):1032.

28.   Schieffer KM, Chuang CH, Connor J, Pawelczyk JA, Sekhar DL. Association of Iron Deficiency Anemia With Hearing Loss in US Adults. *JAMA Otolaryngol Head Neck Surg.* Apr 1 2017;143(4):350-354.

29.   Crosby WH. Whatever became of chlorosis? *Jama.* May 22-29 1987;257(20):2799-2800.

30.   Pawlak R, Berger J, Hines I. Iron Status of Vegetarian Adults: A Review of Literature. *Am J Lifestyle Med.* 2016;12(6):486-498.

31.   U.S. DEPARTMENT OF AGRICULTURE. https://fdc.nal.usda.gov/index.html. Accessed May, 2021.

32.   Stoffel NU, Zeder C, Brittenham GM, Moretti D, Zimmermann MB. Iron absorption from supplements is greater with alternate day than with consecutive day dosing in iron-deficient anemic women. *Haematologica.* May 2020;105(5):1232-1239.

33.   Stoffel NU, Cercamondi CI, Brittenham G, et al. Iron absorption from oral iron supplements given on consecutive versus alternate days and as single morning doses versus twice-daily split dosing in iron-depleted women: two open-label, randomised controlled trials. *Lancet Haematol.* Nov 2017;4(11):e524-e533.

34.   Ferrer-Barceló L, Sanchis Artero L, Sempere García-Argüelles J, et al. Randomised clinical trial: intravenous vs oral iron for the treatment of anaemia after acute gastrointestinal bleeding. *Aliment Pharmacol Ther.* Aug 2019;50(3):258-268.

35.   Block GA, Fishbane S, Rodriguez M, et al. A 12-week, double-blind, placebo-controlled trial of ferric citrate for the treatment of iron deficiency anemia and reduction of serum phosphate in patients with CKD Stages 3-5. *Am J Kidney Dis.* May 2015;65(5):728-736.

36.   Elstrott B, Khan L, Olson S, Raghunathan V, DeLoughery T, Shatzel JJ. The role of iron repletion in adult iron deficiency anemia and other diseases. *Eur J Haematol.* Mar 2020;104(3):153-161.

37.   Adkinson NF, Strauss WE, Macdougall IC, et al. Comparative safety of intravenous ferumoxytol versus ferric carboxymaltose in iron deficiency anemia: A randomized trial. *Am J Hematol.* May 2018;93(5):683-690.

38.   McLoughlin G. Intermittent iron supplementation for reducing anaemia and its associated impairments in adolescent and adult menstruating women. *Int J Evid Based Healthc.* Jun 2020;18(2):274-275.

39.   Pfeiffer CM, Sternberg MR, Schleicher RL, Haynes BM, Rybak ME, Pirkle JL. The CDC's Second National Report on Biochemical Indicators of Diet and Nutrition in the U.S. Population is a valuable tool for researchers and policy makers. *J Nutr.* Jun 2013;143(6):938s-947s.

40.   Ponikowski P, Kirwan BA, Anker SD, et al. Ferric carboxymaltose for iron deficiency at discharge after acute heart failure: a multicentre, double-blind, randomised, controlled trial. *Lancet.* Dec 12 2020;396(10266):1895-1904.

41.   Anker SD, Comin Colet J, Filippatos G, et al. Ferric carboxymaltose in patients with heart failure and iron deficiency. *N Engl J Med.* Dec 17 2009;361(25):2436-2448.

42.   Bothwell TH. Iron requirements in pregnancy and strategies to meet them. *Am J Clin Nutr.* Jul 2000;72(1 Suppl):257s-264s.

ABOUT THE AUTHOR

Dr. Shatzel received his medical degree from the University at Buffalo School of Medicine and Biomedical Sciences. He went on to do Residency in Internal Medicine at Dartmouth College and Fellowship in Hematology and Medical Oncology at Oregon Health & Science University. He currently lives in Portland, Oregon where he is an Assistant Professor of Hematology-Oncology and Biomedical Engineering at Oregon Health & Science University.